Intermittent Fasting

Simple, But Effective Dieting to Lose Weight and Live Longer

Michael Wease

Introduction

I want to thank you and congratulate you for purchasing the book, *"Intermittent fasting"*.

This book has lots of actionable information on how to practice intermittent fasting to lose weight and realize many other benefits you never thought were possible.

If there is any logical way to lose weight, it is through not eating. Why is that so? Well, because many of the dieting approaches you see today all have one goal; to reduce your calorie/carbohydrate intake so as to create the needed calorie deficit to push your body to start burning stored fats for energy.

So if you could just not eat, you can be assured of losing weight because your body would be forced to use up any stored energy i.e. fats for weight loss. There is one problem though; you cannot fast forever as your body needs nutrients to function well - you would die if you stayed for an extended period without food!

What you might wonder is; is there a way you can model that without putting your health and life at risk? Well, there is and that is through intermittent fasting. With intermittent fasting, you don't exactly live without food; you simply schedule your meals so that you eat at certain times and not eat at certain times. And in the end, you are assured of effortless weight loss.

If you are wondering how you can lose weight effortlessly with intermittent fasting, this book has all the information you need to realize effortless maximum weight loss. In this book, you will discover what intermittent fasting is all about, the science behind intermittent fasting, how it works, and how to start following intermittent fasting for effortless weight loss.

If you've been following weight loss regimes that promised a lot only to under-deliver, let this be the last time you are trying to lose weight because with everything you will learn here, if implemented, you can be sure of losing weight effortlessly and keeping it off for good.

Thanks again for downloading this book. I hope you enjoy it!

Table of Contents

Before we learn the specifics of intermittent fasting, it is essential that you have a good understanding of what intermittent fasting is all about and how it works. Let's discuss that.

Intermittent Fasting: The Basics

What Is It?

Intermittent fasting is not a diet but a type of eating pattern where you alternate between periods of fasting and eating. This eating pattern doesn't exactly specify what types of foods to be eaten (or even the amount); just when to eat them. It is as simple as that; you could continue eating whatever it is you've always been eating; all you have to do is to change when you eat. This makes it really easy to follow.

Well, you just don't change your eating time to any time you wish; there are some guidelines that you ought to follow when deciding when you can eat and when you should not be eating. Let me explain:

How Intermittent Fasting Works

For you to understand how intermittent fasting works, it is important to understand how the body processes the food you eat.

When you eat (assuming that you follow the USDA's food pyramid, which entails high carb, minimal fat and moderate protein intake), the body goes into a fed state i.e. a state in which the body has high levels of various nutrients in the bloodstream. The fed state lasts for about 3-5 hours after which your body goes into a post-absorptive state where nothing is being digested although the levels of insulin are still high in the blood. This is the time the cells are taking up any remaining blood glucose for use or storage. During this period (the fed state and post absorptive state, the body is actively digesting everything you've eaten so that some can be absorbed into the bloodstream for transportation to different parts of the body where the cells in various parts use them for energy. After the food is absorbed and is in the bloodstream for transportation to different parts of the body, one challenge arises though; the cells don't have their own mechanism for absorbing glucose from the bloodstream. In fact, they can only do that with the aid of insulin, a hormone secreted by the pancreas in response to rising blood glucose concentrations. The purpose of insulin is simple; to 'open the gates' to the cells so that they can take up the glucose in the bloodstream in order to maintain a healthy level of blood glucose concentration. This essentially means that even if there is an excess of blood glucose (after the fed state), the presence of insulin in the bloodstream keeps the 'doors' open so that the cells take up more glucose. They don't use everything though; the excess glucose is first converted into glycogen, which is then stored in the liver. Glycogen is like an emergency/backup source of energy, which kicks in when glucose levels in the blood are low for an extended period. But the glycogen stores are limited; they can only take about 2000kcal of energy at any given time. So if there is still an excess of glucose available for the cells, it is converted into fatty acids and glycerol, which are then stored in the various fat stores around the body e.g. around organs, under the skin etc. The thing is; the presence of insulin in the bloodstream tends to promote fat storage and inhibits fat burning.

The entire process i.e. being in the fed state (up to the time the body no longer has any glucose which needs to be used up in the bloodstream) takes about 10-12 hours after you've had your meal. If you don't take any more food, this is when you start entering the fasted state, a state where the body has no more glucose in the bloodstream but is 'hungry' for nutrients. What does it do? Well, it goes to its backup power source i.e. glycogen, which it converts into glucose for use in different body processes with the help of glucagon (another hormone secreted by the pancreas) in the liver. At this time, the body doesn't just break down glycogen exclusively; it starts loosening up its grip on other energy stores e.g. the fat stores so that they can be burned to fuel different body processes. This means when you are in a fasted state (i.e. after 12-14 hours from your last meal), you can be sure of losing weight without struggle. The goal of intermittent fasting is to induce the fasted state by spacing meals in a manner that you get to a fasted state every single day so as to push your body to a point of starting to burn glycogen (and perhaps deplete it a little) so that it can start burning more stored fat for energy.

The problem with many of us is that we hardly get to the fasted state; we are very used to eating breakfast, lunch and dinner in some predetermined structure. The challenge though is that this 'structure' hardly gets us into a fasted state. In fact, we are always in the fed state, as many of us eat many meals about 4-5 hours apart. Obviously, this results to a nutrient overload and always keeps us in the fed state because this essentially keeps the body in the fed state. It is only after dinner when we try to get to the fasted state while we are asleep. But given that many of us take breakfast quite early and delay our dinner time, we hardly really 'get there'.

Do you know that this has great adverse effects on your body? Well, let me explain:

As you already know, most of the time, our bodies are in the fed state and not the fasted state making our cells more adopted to burning glucose instead of fat for energy. This simply means that normally, the levels of insulin are always high. There is a problem though; with insulin levels always high, the cells start becoming more 'dump/blind' to the signals of insulin such that more insulin is required to trigger the cells to open up to take up glucose. This is referred to as insulin resistance. In such a state, the body is always burning glucose and rarely ever burns fat (the presence of insulin has fat burning inhibitory properties) and when the glucose is depleted, the body doesn't move to the fasted stage; instead, it gets hungry for more glucose. This is because the body has less capacity to mobilize and burn fat for energy. So you can picture the cravings and the excess fat storage that comes with insulin resistance.

The secret to weight loss is in structuring your meals in a manner that ensures you get your 12-14 hours minimum from the time you had your last meal to the next. The rest of the hours i.e. 12-10 hours are really up to you; eat whatever you want but just don't overindulge! With fasting, this process goes on reverse. When you don't eat for an extended period, the levels of insulin fall as a result of falling blood glucose levels, which signals the body to burn stored energy (glycogen and fats) since no more is coming in. This brings about weight loss in the long term.

From the above explanation, it is clear that the period within which you stay without food ought to start from about 12-14 hours (not less). If you want to fast for longer, you are free to do that; this brings about fasted effects of fasting because you get to use more of the stored fats for energy. The feeding window therefore is within 10-8 hours or less (not more).

Note: You can increase the fasting hours to achieve greater benefits. To make things easier for you, you can follow different intermittent fasting protocols, which we will discuss later.

So how exactly does intermittent fasting result to weight loss? Well, there are different explanations to this:

1: You effectively create a calorie deficit when you fast.

2: You ultimately are likely to consume fewer calories within the feeding window, something which will definitely create the much needed calorie deficit for weight loss

3: You enhance your metabolism with intermittent fasting.

While the first two points look somewhat straightforward, the 3rd point might not be so straightforward. We will discuss how intermittent fasting affects your metabolism next.

How Intermittent Fasting Affects Your Metabolism

Most people have the idea that skipping meals leads to a slow metabolic rate because your body will need to preserve as much energy as it can. Well, it is true that extremely long periods without food can lead to a slower metabolism but studies have also shown that fasting for short periods actually increases your metabolism and not slow it down. One study published in NCBI conducted on 11 healthy men proved that a 3 day fast increased their metabolism by a notable 14%!

This was thought to be because of the rise of the hormone known as norepinephrine, which promotes the burning of fat. This hormone is a stress hormone that improves attention and alertness and has a number of other effects on the body. One of them is instructing the body's fat cells to release fatty acids. The more the norepinephrine is in your bloodstream, the larger the amounts of fatty acids that are availed for your body to burn.

Other ways that intermittent fasting impacts your metabolism positively include the following:

1: Eliminating wastes

It is normal for toxins to accumulate in your system during ordinary drinking and eating. During intermittent fasting, your body is able to eliminate those toxins and wastes (as you get to regularly clear your digestive system) hence cleansing your internal organs. This in turn increases your metabolism as there are no toxins to hinder digestion.

As you cut down on particular foods at particular times during intermittent fasting, your system gets a window where it can cleanse itself and remove toxins and wastes. So when you get to eat, your body doesn't have to use energy for both digestion and removing toxins- it can fully focus on digestion and other processes in the system.

Intermittent fasting also regulates digestion. Slow digestion negatively affects your body's ability to break down food and burn fat. A clear bowel is a healthy bowel and on a fast, your body has less to digest thus reducing the work that the system has to carry out. This promotes healthy bowel and metabolic function.

2: Trains the body to burn fat

When you are fasting, your body is temporarily deprived of the normal sugars that it is usually used to burning for fuel- the sugars would be used as the primary source of fuel. This forces your body to turn on the fat burning metabolism to meet its energy requirements.

This ensures you burn fat in the short term (during your fast) and also resets your body to depend more on fat for energy during normal eating (as the body will be expecting less food). This means that your metabolism will improve from glucose burning to fat burning.

3: Regulates blood sugar

Mostly people associate eating with gnawing feelings of deep hunger. But the thing is; hunger is majorly caused by shifts in blood sugar levels. With intermittent fasting, your body burns fat (and not sugars) at a steady rate hence keeping your hunger under control since there is no frequent conversion and stagnation of blood sugars in the system. Also, as your body burns fat for energy, this leaves behind a satiating feeling, which you cannot experience if you are in the fed state where blood glucose levels are high.

This means that the level of insulin in the system is also reduced, a phenomenon that lowers the risk of insulin resistance (where insulin becomes ineffective) making sure that digestion and metabolism in general, stays perfect.

4: Better eating habits

Fasting also certainly changes your attitude towards food in that you become less dependent on it and in turn gain more clarity about what you will be eating and what's best for you. Once you know what's necessary for your body for optimum function, you will be led to eating right, which will energize your metabolism. For instance, eating right could mean that you incorporate more fiber, which leads to easier digestion of foods.

5: Slowing down of the aging process

When you give your body a rest from normal digestion through fasting, your body can be able to slow down aging, as it has less overall work to perform. Generally, this gives your digestive system a break, as you will be eating less. This can boost your metabolism so that more fat is burned down, which leads to inevitable weight loss.

This is really significant because one of the major consequences of aging is a slower metabolism. The younger your body stays, the more efficient and faster your metabolism will be.

With that understanding, I know you might now be wondering; so how exactly can you follow intermittent fasting? We will discuss the different intermittent fasting protocols next.

The Types of Intermittent Fasting

How you want to follow your intermittent fasting totally depends on you- on the basis of time, food portions and length of fast. But there are a number of different types of intermittent fasting that can narrow down your options- feel free to go with the one that best suits your interests:

Alternate-Day Fasting

Coined by: James Johnson M.D

Best suited for: Serious dieters that have a defined goal weight

How it works

This type of fasting, also known as Up day Down Day diet, means fasting every other day. There can be all sorts of variations for this type of fast. For instance, one most common variations allows around 500 calories during the fast days whereas others nothing at all (during the fast days).

It could also be as simple as eating very little during the fast days and then eating like you normally do the next day. Very little means 1/5 of what you normally eat. For instance, if you normally eat 2000 calories a day, then on the fast days, you should only have 400 calories.

Tip: A full 24 hour fast every other day seems a bit hard so if you are a beginner, it would be best to steer clear of the Alternate day fasting method first.

The pros

This method is fully based around weight loss (through cutting back on calories) so if that's your goal then it will work perfectly for you.

The cons

You might find it a bit difficult to work out on the low calorie days- opt to keep work outs less strenuous during these days and save the harder sessions for normal days.

Tip: This method is easy to follow but it is prone to binging during the normal days. The best way to avoid this is by planning your meals ahead and knowing what you are eating.

The 16/8 Method

Coined by: Martin Berkhan

Best suited for: Focused gym-goers that want to build muscle and lose body fat. It is also suitable if you that have some sort of flexibility at work (or school) such that you can be able to easily plan for your meals and work outs.

This method of intermittent fasting, also known as Leangains Protocol, involves fasting for around 14 to 16 hours each day and restricting your 'eating window' to around 8 to 10 hours (the period where you can have your meals). During the eating window, you can fit in 2, 3 or even more meals.

This method can be as simple as avoiding meals after dinner and skipping breakfast. For example, if you have dinner at around 8 pm and then do not eat anything until 12 noon then you are basically fasting for 16 hours a day. The recommended fast time for women is 14 to 15 hours as slightly shorter fasts have proved to work better for them.

If you are a mad breakfast lover and you tend to get hungry in the morning then this will take a bit of time to adjust. During the fast, you can drink coffee, water or other non caloric beverages to help reduce hunger.

As much as this schedule is easily adaptable to anyone's life style, it is important to maintain a constant feeding window time or else your hormones can get thrown off making sticking to the diet even harder- according to Berkhan.

A rough idea of what to eat:

What you eat on the feeding window depends on when you work out. On the days you exercise, carbs consumption is more important than fat- since the carbs will be used up during your work out. On the rest days, fat consumption should be higher. Protein consumption should be relatively high each day- though it varies with gender, goals, age, activity levels and body fat. To be more specific:

During work out days- break your fast with veggies, meat and a fruit. If you plan to work out anytime soon after the meal then toss in a few carbs from starch- e.g. whole grain bread or potatoes. Remember though not to stuff yourself- make it a medium sized meal. You should train within three hours after taking the meal and then have larger meal after the work out where you add more complex carbs- you can even have a treat as dessert as long as it is not too high in fat and large in size. An example of such is low fat ice cream and sorbet and not treats such as a birthday cake.

On the rest days- you should eat way less calories than during the work outs. Cut down on your carbs intake and feast more on fibrous veggies, meat and fruit; your first meal during the feeding period should be the largest contrary to during the work out days where the after- work out meal is the largest. 'Largest' doesn't have to really be in terms of volume- ideally 40% of your caloric intake in the meal should be from proteins. If the meat is fatty (like salmon and ground beef) then the better it is.

For the last meal of the day- include a protein that is slow digesting such as cottage cheese or egg protein. Fish or meat is also just fine as long as you supplement it with fiber or veggies. This will ensure that you are kept full all through the fast and that your body has an adequate supply of amino acids up to the next meal.

Also, it is important that during the fast you get your macros from healthy foods as this won't work if you consume loads of junk food and excess calories. Give a priority to whole and unprocessed foods over liquid and overly processed foods- unless you have to compromise. For instance, you might not have time to eat a meal let alone prepare it. In such a case, you can have a meal replacement bar or a protein shake.

This type of intermittent fasting can be said to be the most 'natural' way to do it- but who I'm I to judge!

The pros

For most people, the best part of this method is that the meal frequency is irrelevant as you can eat whenever you want during the feeding window. And since the meals are larger (though infrequent) you get to be fuller for longer.

Also, this method is mostly preferred because of its state-of-the-art level of hormonal control. While something like the alternate day fasting will give you such benefits, it is not for daily practice. The Leangains on the other hand means that you get to have a daily increase in the levels of growth hormone which leads to greater effects.

To add on to that, practicing daily means that you are eating the same way each day meaning that you don't experience fluctuations in hunger since your body is already used to that kind of eating.

The Cons

Although there is flexibility on the case of when you can eat, the 16/8 method has a few specific guidelines on what you should eat especially when working out is concerned. This can make it a bit difficult to follow the protocols and determine when to eat and when to fast.

Eat-Stop-Eat

Coined by: Brad Pilon

Best for: Healthy eaters seeking for an extra boost

This method of intermittent fasting involves full 24 hour fasts either once or twice in a week. When you fast from dinner on one day to dinner the next day then you would have done an Eat-Stop-Eat fast. You can also make it a breakfast to breakfast fast or a lunch to lunch fast- as long as you have done full 24 hours then you are good. The main rationale about this method is reducing your overall caloric intake without necessarily limiting what you are able to eat. Incorporating regular workouts with this method will make reaching your goals faster and easier if improved body composition and weight loss are the goals.

Moreover, if your main aim of doing this kind of fast is to lose weight, then it is advisable to eat normally during the feeding periods- in other words, you should eat how you would have eaten if you were not fasting. Make sure that you keep yourself occupied during the fast to avoid eating. You can also sleep and make sure to get enough liquids.

Coffee, water and other non caloric beverages are allowed when fasting although no solid food should be consumed.

The pros

I know a 24 hour fast can seem like a long time, to go without eating but the good thing is that you don't have to dive all in at once. You can go for as long as you can without food and then increase the time bit by bit.

There also no forbidden foods in this type of intermittent fasting and also no counting calories and other restrictions which makes it easier to follow. You still need to eat like an adult- in moderation.

It is also really hard to screw up with a 24-hour fast. The only rule is to not eat for 24 hours- from 8pm to 8pm. It is also easily adaptable to any life style as you can choose a feeding time that is most convenient for you.

The Cons

The downside about this fast it is that for most people, it can be a bit challenging to go for a full 24 hours without food- hence the advice to start small and work your way to the top. Most people have difficulty going for long periods without food with complaints such as fatigue, headaches and feeling cranky- but these effects diminish over time.

The long fast can also make binging more tempting after a fast is over. This needs self control which, sorry to say, some people lack.

The Warrior Diet

Coined by: Ori Hofmekler

Best for: The devoted- those people who like following rules

This is one of the most popular type of intermittent fasting that involves eating raw vegetables and fruits during the day and then eating a huge meal during the night (like a warrior). You basically get to 'feast' at night within an eating window of 4 hours and 'fast' all day.

What you eat and when you eat it is key in this method. This diet insists on food choices that are really similar to the paleo diet (another reason for the name) -foods that are whole and unprocessed resembling how they actually looked like in nature. The idea here is to feed the body the nutrients that it needs in accordance to the circadian rhythms and for the reason that our species are nightly eaters that are programmed to eat at night.

The fasting phase of this method is all about under eating as during the 20 hours you can eat a few servings of veggies, fresh juice and a bit of protein if desired. This is intended to maximize the 'fight or flight' response of the Sympathetic Nervous System which is intended to stimulate fat burning, promote alertness and boost energy.

On the other hand, the 4 hour window when you can eat, regarded as the overeating phase, is meant to be at night to maximize the ability of the Parasympathetic nervous system to assist the body to recuperate by promoting calm relaxation while letting the body use the nutrients taken in for growth and repair. Eating during the day can also assist the body to produce hormones and burn fat during daytime- according to Hofmekler. You also have to eat specific foods during the eating window- ideally start with veggies, protein and fat. If you are still hungry after this then you can have a bit of carbs.

The pros

Many people love this fasting method given that it allows you to have small snacks which make it really easier to get through it. The small snacks can lead to increased energy levels which will get you through the day.

The cons

Although having a few snacks is better than eating nothing, the guidelines of what you need to eat and when to eat them can be a bit difficult to stick to in the long run.

For some people, this method interferes with social gatherings as it can be tricky to follow the strict meal plan and schedule during such gatherings.

Furthermore, this can be difficult to practice for the people who prefer not to eat huge meals late at night.

The 5:2 Method

Coined by: Michael Mosley

Best for: Healthy eaters with less time on their hands for a strict meal schedule

This diet is characterized by normal eating for 5 days of the week then limiting your calories to 500 to 600 on the rest of the 2 days of the week. This method, popularized by the British doctor Michael Mosley, is also known as the Fast diet.

The method requires women to consume 500 calories during the fast days and men 600 calories on the fasting days. The days don't have to be consequent to each other. For instance, you can eat normally on all the days of the week except on Thursday and Monday where you have 2 or 3 small meals (ideally 250 calories each for women and 300 for men) and then for the rest of the days you eat normally. You can choose any 2 days of the week that are most suitable to you provided that you have at least one day when you are not fasting in between the days that you are fasting.

It is important to keep in mind that eating 'normally' doesn't really mean you are free to eat anything you want. If you eat tons of junk food then most likely you won't lose any weight- or even worse you may put on a few pounds.

Although there are no rules on what you can eat on the fast days, most people function quite well by starting off with a small breakfast while others prefer to start eating as late as possible.

There are generally 2 meal patterns here for the fast days that are commonly used:

Three small meals: inclusive of breakfast, lunch and dinner

Two slightly bigger meals: consists of only lunch and dinner

As you know, your caloric budget is limited so you have to make wise decisions. Focus on nutritious high protein, high fiber foods that are low in calories and will keep you full. Soups are a great example. Other examples are veggies, cauliflower rice, natural yogurt with some berries, baked or boiled eggs, lean meat or grilled fish, black coffee, tea etc.

The pros

The 5:2 diet causes weight loss just as calorie restriction does. The diet is also really effective at reducing the levels of insulin and improving insulin sensitivity (once you adhere to avoiding junk food during the fast and non fast days).

The cons

Making the wrong food choices during the fast days can lead to exceeding the calorie requirement which will beat the purpose of the method.

Spontaneous Meal Skipping

As I mentioned earlier, intermittent fasting is all about choice. You don't really need to follow a defined fasting plan to get the benefits of this method. This option gives you the chance to skip meals when it is most convenient to you- say when you are too busy to cook and eat or when you just don't feel hungry.

Trust me, it is a myth that people have to eat after every few hours or else they will lose muscle or go to 'starvation mode'. You body is essentially equipped to handle extended courses of famine let alone skipping a few meals from time to time. So if you find that you are not hungry during a specific meal then don't force yourself; skip it and wait until the next meals. Just ensure you eat healthy when it comes to the next meal.

Now that you have an understanding of what intermittent fasting is all about, our next chapter will focus entirely on easing into intermittent fasting.

How to Gradually Transition into Intermittent Fasting

Everything takes a bit if time and getting used to. You can't possibly wake up one day and not eat for 14 straight hours when you never have before. Slow steps are recommended if you are planning to incorporate intermittent fasting as part of your life style. Follow the following ideas to help you ease into intermittent fasting:

Set your goal

Before anything else, you should determine what exactly you want to achieve through intermittent fasting. This can give you added mental strength if you will need it. Some of the possible specific intermittent fasting goals you can set are:

- Reducing the time spent eating- this prevents excessive body weight gain and possible liver damage. If you aim to reduce the time you spend eating, then you can try out the warrior diet (where you eat nothing (or raw fruits and veggies) during the day and one meal at night or the 16/8 method.

- Extending your lifetime expectancy by reducing overall body fat and cholesterol levels- intermittent fasting helps in lowering the blood sugar and blood pressure levels through reduction of fat and cholesterol in the body. In this case, any method of intermittent fasting can work for you as long as you accompany it with low carb eating. Even when you do have carbs, avoid processed and refined ones. Opt for more natural ones such as sweet potatoes and whole grains.

- Simply losing body fat and weight loss- as already ascertained, intermittent fasting is a great way to lose weight. The choice of the method in this case lies in your hands.

- Relieving inflammation in your body- time restricted feeding increases bile acid production which improves adipose tissue homeostasis and in the end alleviates inflammation. Intermittent fasting is all about time restricted feeding so also in this case you can go with any method. But also, during the feeding, make sure you avoid foods that cause inflammation such as dairy, refined flour and vegetable oils.

- Other goals which could work perfectly with any kind of intermittent fasting are raising mass of organ, bone and muscle (through increasing the growth hormone levels), enhancing focus and alertness (through accelerating nor-epinephrine levels) and raising your metabolism.

Start intermittent fasting

So how do you start? It is really simple actually. If you decide on the 16/8 method, just make lunch your first meal on the 1st day regardless of when you ate dinner. In fact, this method is awesome for beginners as most of the fast time you will be asleep making it less agonizing. If you were used to feeding your body every 3 hours then you are bound to feel hungry the first few days of trying fasting.

Remember to go at it gradually; going all in is a recipe for failure as it will be too much of a drastic change for your body to handle- if you have never fasted before.

Sleep as part of your fast and always keep yourself busy when awake

When you start fasting, it will feel natural to look forward to when you will be having later on. But you have to realize that you can't base your life on thinking about what to eat next. See it as part of how you normally do things and continue your routine as usual. Take a nap when you feel overwhelmed.

When it comes to the feasting time then eat! Try and eat a bit healthy and don't go too low on fats and carbs- as you will get feelings of being deprived and unsatisfied.

Allow your system to detox as you ease into the fast

It is important to reduce the irritating symptoms of toxicity by letting your system to naturally detox to make the fast easier for you. Ease into the fast by altering your diet first to kick out processed foods- granola bars, proteins bars, processed meat, soda, you name it. Once your system is clear, you will have an easier time getting into your fast and breaking your fast as you won't have fluctuating insulin levels which are the cause of hunger (if you can remember).

Wisely choose your last non-fasting meal

You should always opt for more fresh fruits and veggies. When starting intermittent fasting, most people binge a little which is not advisable as it means that most of the fast time will be spent digesting food and less of the time in the fasting adapted stage.

Avoid eating huge amounts of carbs and sugars especially during the last feeding period as this will make you hungrier way earlier into your fast because of the high 'sugar rush' which will be followed by a low sugar crash.

Is there a way to keep off the hunger pangs? Let's briefly discuss that:

Tips to Fight Off Hunger During the Fasting Period

As long as you are human and you are trying out intermittent fasting, then you are bound to feel hungry at one point or another. Some of the ways to keep the hunger in control are:

Drinking lots of water

Aside from being the healthiest and easiest method of fighting hunger, staying well hydrated can make fasting much easier to get thorough. Most of the time, thirst is confused for hunger so anytime you feel hungry, just gobble down a glass of water. Keep this in mind as it will be your number 1 way to stave off hunger.

Have a cup of coffee or organic tea

Other than water, there are other fluids that can help keep the hunger as far from you as possible. Caffeine and other stimulants of the nervous system work as appetite suppressants; consumption of coffee has been proven to stimulate the release of the hormone cholecystokinin (CCK) which is one of the hormones released after eating that gives us a calm feeling. This hormone makes us full and takes away the feelings of eating.

Also, a simple cup of tea or coffee can hydrate your system and boost your energy levels with a bonus of delivering a wave of antioxidants. Start your day with a cup of either (tea or coffee) or have a cup whenever you feel hunger kicking in.

Meditation

Meditation helps you to relax, sit still and control how you think- this can help control anxiety and stress. Although this is not the easiest way to control hunger, meditation works miracles over time. As you get better at it, you will learn to control hunger and even perhaps embrace it.

 Meditating will help you avoid the temptations of breaking a fast as you get to think clearly of what you want and the benefits you will get after sticking to the fast.

Engage in some short and intense exercise

Engaging in intervals of short and intense exercise during the fasting period is a sure way to keep your mind from focusing on hunger. Intense exercise such as sprinting or lifting weights also blasts fats and boosts muscles and more importantly, directly suppresses appetite.

Different types of exercises can lead to production or reduction of different kinds of appetite suppressing hormones. For instance, aerobics are known to suppress a hormone known as ghrelin, which increases appetite and increases the production of peptide YY which decrease appetite- 20 to 30 minutes of such exercise when you are about to finish your fast is ideal.

If you are not at work, then go crazy on household chores

If your fast day falls on a day when you are not at work (or you work at home but you aren't working for the day) then household chores will do the trick when it comes to fighting off hunger.

Cleaning or gardening will keep you focused on something else other than food and also help you have a more organized and cleaner yard. You can also take this advantage and grow your own food. Homegrown foods are the best way to ensure you eat healthy and avoid any unknown toxins.

Do any pending work related tasks

Do you know that report or project that you have been putting off or all those unread emails that are packed in your inbox? This is the great opportunity to work on them. Ensure that your fast is productive and that you don't spend the whole day obsessing over your next meal.

When you are not eating, base your focus on something else productive- it could be school work, job related tasks or social related activities. The busier you are, the more successful your fast will be.

Play some sports or engage in a hobby

Any type of physical activity that you engage in is going to have a positive impact on your fast- just as long as you keep it moderate. If you have favorite sport such as basket ball or tennis or any other type of physical hobby such as boxing then engage in it during the fasting period.

This is a great way to trick your body into both exercise and fasting since your mind is fully focused on the activity and not the fasting or exercising. This is because it is something you enjoy and you consider it as play.

Take a walk

Taking brisk walks increases fat burning effects of a fast. A brisk walk also nourishes a healthy heart and promotes general health. Combining a fast and a brisk walk could be the best thing you could do for your body.

Like other kinds of exercise, a brisk walk can keep your hunger in control. It can do this by first of all providing a fun distraction and motivating the body to start burning stored fat for energy.

You can take your dog out for a walk, go out to buy groceries or if it's in the morning you can walk to work instead of taking the bus.

Munch on some live foods

This should be the last option for controlling hunger. If you find out that you simply cant 100% control your hunger and you really need to eat then the best option is to enter into a 'controlled fast'- this is similar to the under eating phase of the warrior diet.

Here, you will have to eat very lightly during the fast- foods that have the lowest glycemic index (those that have the least impact on your blood sugar levels). The foods should only be live veggies and fruits- they should not be cooked at all. Also, make sure to keep the servings small.

Other Tips to Make Intermittent Fasting Successful

Rewire how you think: think of fasting more as a break from eating rather than a moment of deprivation. Take it as a way to break the routine of worrying about what to eat and when you will eat it next. This will help you stick to fasting for a long term.

Over commit: it might seem as a not- so- good idea but starting fasting when you are busy is the best way to do it. If you do it while you have the whole day to sit on the couch, the chances of snacking are pretty high.

Hit the gym: consistent exercise paired with intermittent fasting ensures better results. You don't have to go all out- something as basic as a full body strength training routine for 2 to 3 times a week is enough.

Give it a minimum of 3 weeks: if you haven't given intermittent fasting at least 3 weeks then you don't have the right to give up. After this then you can determine if the method is for you as you would have given it enough time to adapt. Check your progress on your goal (e.g. if it is weight loss, see how much you've lost so far) and assess how you feel about the whole thing.

Don't tell people you are fasting: as much as intermittent fasting is becoming popular in the health and fitness world, there are still a great number of skeptics and uneducated people who have no idea about the perks of the fast. Some people might think that you are trying to starve yourself while others might tell you that you are outright crazy for even trying it.

It is advisable to keep it to yourself more so when you are starting. We all know that words sting and you might even end up quitting.

Intermittent Fasting As a Lifestyle

If you want to stick to intermittent fasting for life, then you must not view it as a diet but as a life style. This will require you to reevaluate your eating choices even before beginning the fast so that when you begin, you are sure that you won't be going back. For example, if you use regular vegetable oil then it is time to replace it with healthy oils such as coconut oil and olive oil. If you tend to eat processed carbs then it is time to replace them with healthy whole unprocessed carbs- e.g. zucchini noodles in place of pasta.

The idea here is to embrace the diet and the fact that your body will be a full on fat burning means that new carbs won't be required for body fuel. It will typically take a few weeks for this to happen but once it does, cravings for unhealthy carbs will be out of the picture and incorporating this diet into your life will be as easy as ABC.

If you are going to live the ultimate intermittent fasting lifestyle then:

The best way to include Intermittent Fasting into your life style is by delaying your breakfast slowly by slowly- delay by an hour then another hour the next day and so on. Take an hour to shower, an hour to do your chores, an hour to get to work- just take an hour from any activity that you engage in the morning that you see best fit until you get to a time that you can live with.

Do not use fasting as an excuse to eat junk- calories are different. 100 calories of broccoli are not the same as 100 calories of a snicker bar. When you find yourself cheating then get real with yourself. Keep the carbs for before work outs and fill yourself up with meats and veggies.

Stick to the method that you are most comfortable with- as discussed, there are a number of ways to do intermittent fasting. Play around with all of them and get what suits you best. Make sure you actually try out all methods- you might be surprised which will be easiest to follow. In order to make something part of your lifestyle, you need to be fully comfortable with it. Intermittent fasting is no different.

Conclusion

We have come to the end of the book. Thank you for reading and congratulations for reading until the end.

I hope the book has opened your eyes to the endless ways through which intermittent fasting can transform your life and how to use it to realize the benefits.

If you found the book valuable, can you recommend it to others? One way to do that is to post a review on Amazon. It'd be greatly appreciated!

Thank you and good luck!

79459682R00024

Made in the USA
San Bernardino, CA
14 June 2018